FIX

AND

FIT

Weight loss, get your body in place or costume just the way you love it.

Roy B. Williams

CONTENTS

Chapter 4

LIVING A NORMAL LIFE AND KEEPING A HEALTHY WEIGHT

Chapter 5

INCREASING ENERGY

Chapter 6

CONCLUSION

INTRODUCTION

Living a happy life requires losing weight, but it's not always as simple as many think it will be! It needs the highest commitment, consistency, and balance, which is why this trip will be so rewarding in the end! Of course, maintaining your allocated diet programs, exercise routines, or training demands ongoing motivation as well!

It is possible, but whether you choose to make it happen is entirely up to you. You will lose weight if you put in the effort.

Forgetting who you are and remembering who you want to be is the most exciting aspect of getting it done.

Put an end to the notion that you should lose weight and become skinny. Put an end to your desire to be curvy. Just begin to consider your health. It's not necessary to wait until you're now skinny before declaring your mission successful. No. It's okay as long as there is a deduction, as long as you can now begin performing those things that previously seemed unattainable to you, and you feel delighted.

Chapter 1

QUICKLY LOSING STUBBORN FAT AND WEIGHT

You can't preserve a healthy weight because of just following certain guidelines, programs, or diet plans. Rather, it only encloses a way of life for stress reduction, frequent exercise, and healthy eating habits.

The ones who engage in the gradual process of losing weight (between 1 and 2 pounds per week) have a better chance of keeping it off than those who lose weight abruptly.

Having proper control of weight loss might be troubled by settings, environments, sleep, age, genetics, diseases, medications, and diseases. Speak with your healthcare professional if you are worried about your weight or have concerns about your medications.

Getting Going
It takes careful planning to lose weight. Here is a starting point.

Step 1: Commit yourself.
 Write out your motivations for shedding pounds, such as wanting to see your children get married or wanting to feel better in your clothes. Your goals can only be achieved by writing them down. Posting these arguments will act as a daily reminder of your motivation for the shift.

Step 2: Evaluate your current situation.
For a few days, record everything you consume in a food and beverage diary. You can prevent thoughtless consumption by being more conscious of what you eat and drink. Understanding existing routines and pressures can also be accomplished by

keeping track of physical activity, sleep, and emotions. Additionally, it can show you where to start making modifications.

Examine your lifestyle next. Of Course, there are lots of things that may stop you from achieving your weight loss goals. For instance, you find it challenging to stay away from sugary foods especially when you buy them for your kids, or love eating food high in calories, like doughnuts. Consider what you can do to aid in overcoming these obstacles.

Step 3: Make sensible objectives
Prepare a positive plan, follow it up and ensure you monitor your development. Maybe your long-term objectives are to control your high blood pressure and shed 40 pounds. As well as Your short-term intention might just be having a vegetable with dinner or choosing water over sugary drinks to drink.

Concentrate on two or three objectives at once. Effective objectives are:
Specific, realistic, and forgiving (but not ideal)
For instance, the statement "exercise more" is vague. However, being specific and practical, "I will walk

for 15 minutes, three days a week for the first week," is better.

Setting impossible objectives, like shedding 20 pounds in two weeks, might make you feel disappointed and dejected.

Living practically as well includes being ready for a few hiccups here and there. Get back on track as soon as you can after setbacks. Additionally, consider how to avoid failures in similar circumstances in the future.
Remember that everyone is unique, therefore what suits one person may not be suitable for another. Try different sports or exercises like walking, swimming, tennis, or group fitness programs. See what you can fit into your life and that you most love. Long-term commitment to these activities will be simpler.

Even Small Weight Loss Is Beneficial
Significant advantages, including reductions in blood pressure, blood cholesterol, and blood sugar levels, can result in even modest weight loss.

For instance, if you weigh 200 pounds and lose 5% of that weight, you will weigh 190 pounds. Your chance of developing chronic diseases linked to obesity can be reduced by this small weight loss.

Step 4: Locate sources of knowledge and assistance
Welcome friends or relatives who are supportive of you in getting rid of that stubborn fat. Coworkers or neighbors with comparable objectives might exchange healthy cooking tips and organize social exercise events, you may even find it favorable to link up with a group of promotive people who are trying to lose weight or speak with a qualified nutritionist.

Step 5: Continue to keep track of your development
Review your Step 3 objectives again and monitor your development. Do ensure to know which aspect of your plan needs to be adjusted and which ones are working effectively. Again, revisit your goals and come up with something new.
Add a new objective to assist you in continuing down your successful path if you routinely achieve a current one.

Reward your achievements to yourself! Be proud of your accomplishments and acknowledge when you reach your goals. Use non-food incentives like a bouquet, a sports outing with friends, or a little soothing bath instead of food. Rewarding yourself keeps you motivated to maintain your improved health.

A greater risk of diabetes, stroke, and certain types of cancer are among the health hazards associated with being overweight.

Why should I lose weight?

There are various causes for weight loss, including:

1. Enticing: Having the right shape or bodybuilding and not being overly large will make you appear more attractive, fit, or healthy.

2. Self-satisfaction and body image:
Being obese or overweight looks so boring and tiring at times, because you may feel uneasy about the way you look.

3. General well-being: Having a normal weight keeps up perfect general health and fends off conditions like type 2 diabetes.

4. certain circumstances: When a person loses extra weight, for instance, their type 2 diabetes or sleep apnea symptoms may become better or go altogether.

5. Fitness: Participating in an exercise-based weight-loss program is likely helpful to feeling fitter, more energized, and more resilient.

6. Athletic contests: In some sports, like boxing, a competitor may try to maintain their current weight category by exercising self-control.

7. Fertility: Women with obesity and polycystic ovarian syndrome (PCOS) may benefit more from fertility treatment if they lose weight before starting it.

Calories

The maximum calorie consumption one is expected
to take in for weight loss depends on a variety of
factors.
Among these elements are:
wished-for weight loss
ideal weight loss rate
age, sex

For men, the suggested daily caloric intake is as
follows:
Actively involved: 1,800
Present: 2000 to 2200
A person should consume fewer calories than those
indicated above if they want to lose weight.
(Striking that appropriate balance) Keeping up a
balanced, wholesome food is necessary
If at all feasible, a person should consult a dietitian,
nutritionist, or physician before making any dietary
changes.

To maintain optimum health, make sure protein,
carbohydrate, and fat ratios are appropriate.

Although it's known that a lack of adequate nourishment and poor dietary intake is seemingly unavoidable regardless of calories, a meal plan should be balanced in terms of nutrients. Not being extremely happy and full of incentive can likely occur as a result of a poor diet.

It's necessary for one to continuously augment their daily calorie intake after reaching their desired body weight until they reach their "weight maintenance" aim.

Weight management

It's natural and productive to manage your body weight by using a balanced diet and frequent exercise.Catching on to a good Sleeping hour can as well aid someone in managing their weight. According to scientific research, poor sleep may cause cravings, increased appetite, and a decline in the desire to exercise.

Several ways of managing your weight when done reducing. Here are some tips:

Avoid calorie-restrictive diets since they can impede metabolism and change hormones that control appetite. Weight gain may result from this.

Exercise: 200 minutes a week of exercise can aid in maintaining weight loss.

Prefer consuming protein a lot because it helps to feel satisfied and less hungry.

A low-carb diet has been shown in several studies to help people maintain their weight loss after losing it.

Weight and health

According to some experts and medical professionals, diets and weight-loss initiatives may result in more weight gain and worse health. Long-term weight loss was greater in those who had personalized food plans combined with goal-oriented psychotherapy.

Overeating is the primary contributor to obesity, hence it should be addressed as an eating problem. Psychotherapy that supports weight loss can help lessen the negative impacts of problems brought on by conventional diets.

Supplements

Numerous supplements on the market promise to aid with weight loss.
A few of these are:
Products with omega-3s and fish oils
Chitosan is a substance made from shellfish, green tea extract, and various Chinese herbs.
Additionally, evidence indicates that these are ineffective and may cause negative effects.

Considering safety first, ephedra, a former component of certain weight-loss products, is now prohibited.

Natural solutions:

Methods that emphasize both the body and the mind may be beneficial.
Examples comprise:
yogic breathing and eating
In getting the best out of this process it's recommended you reach out to a knowledgeable and

skilled instructor to lead you through these exercises.

Weight loss surgery
A surgical technique for persons whose body mass index is high enough to put them at risk of catastrophic complications is bariatric surgery, sometimes referred to as weight loss surgery.
A doctor might advise bariatric surgery if other weight loss methods have failed.
Either a gastric band or stomach reduction is part of the operation.

In some circumstances, a doctor might advise a particular kind of gastric bypass procedure where the small intestines are diverted to a tiny stomach pouch.
A person's appetite will be significantly reduced after surgery, and they won't be able to digest or absorb food as well as they once could.

When is losing weight bad?
Sometimes, losing weight might lead to issues.

During the interval whereby extra vitality is exhausted and then taken in, weight loss occurs. An unsupportive energy steadiness is what this is. To fill the gap, the body looks for energy reserves, starting with fat.

 Any extra muscle and lean tissue in a person with low body fat will be lost. This could lead to other health problems.

These include:
a higher risk of osteoporosis, lower strength and muscle mass, problems controlling body temperature, and a reduced ability to fight infections. A substantial loss of body mass can be fatal.

A person who is suddenly losing weight should see a doctor if at all possible.

In conclusion, there are several factors to consider when attempting to lose weight, such as age, sex, food, level of activity, and medical conditions.

Health professionals have shown that reducing calories, moving more, eating a balanced diet, and getting adequate sleep can all help people lose weight.

In some circumstances, a person could gain from having surgery to decrease weight, such as bariatric surgery. However, over-losing of weight is wrong and can be harmful to health.

If at all possible, a person should consult a doctor before making changes to their diet or exercise program.

10 suggestions for effective weight loss
Overview: Despite the availability of numerous "fad" diets, maintaining a healthy weight and leading a balanced lifestyle are the keys to good health.
Obesity raises the risk of significant health issues like heart disease, high blood pressure, and type 2 diabetes.
Despite any benefits they may have, crash diets are not a long-term answer. It is crucial to adopt progressive, healthy lifestyle adjustments to lose weight healthily and maintain it over time.

10 recommendations for efficient weight loss
People can lose weight and keep it off by taking a few realistic steps.
These are what they include:
1. Eat a range of colorful, nutrient-rich foods.
Eat a balanced, healthful diet.
Healthy meals and snacks should be the foundation of human diets. Building a meal plan is simple if you make sure that every meal has 50% fruit and vegetables, 25% whole grains, and 25% protein.
Each day, 25 to 30 grams (g) of fiber should be consumed.

Ensure you takeaway trans fats off your meals and shorten saturated fats, which are highly related to the development of coronary heart disease.
People could also consume unsaturated fats such as polyunsaturated fatty acids (PUFA) or monounsaturated fatty acids as an alternative.

The following foods are generally healthy and high in nutrients:
Fresh fruits and vegetables, seafood, lentils, nuts, and whole grains like oats and brown rice are all good options.

Avoid eating the following foods:
fatty red or processed meats, baked goods with extra
sugar, butter, or oils
sliced bread, bagels, and prepared foods
In rare cases, eliminating certain items from the diet
could cause someone to become deficient in some
vital vitamins and minerals. A nutritionist, dietician,
or other healthcare professional can provide advice
on how to get enough nutrients while following a
weight loss program.

2. Record your food and weight
People are considerably more likely to continue to a
weight loss routine if they can gauge their progress
in modest steps and spot visible improvements.

3. Perform frequent physical activity and exercise.
Regular exercisers can lose weight.
Keeping to exercise always is so relevant because it
helps in sustaining good physical and mental health.
Regularly increasing physical activity while being
disciplined and intentional is generally crucial for
weight loss success.
One hour of brisk walking is the recommended
amount of moderate-intensity exercise per day.

People who are not generally active should gradually increase the amount and intensity of their exercise. The best long-term method for ensuring that regular exercise becomes a way of life for them is this one.

In the same way that keeping track of their meals might aid in weight loss, people may experience psychological advantages from doing so. After documenting their food intake and exercise, a person can use a selection of free mobile apps to monitor their calorie balance.

To improve their fitness, a beginner who finds the thought of a full workout intimidating can start by doing the activities below:

leaf-raking, dog-walking, gardening, dancing, outdoor activities, and parking farther from a building's entrance are all examples of activities that involve climbing steps.
Patients with low-risk coronary heart disease are unlikely to require a physical examination before starting an activity program.
But for certain people, especially those who have diabetes, a prior medical examination might be wise.

4. Limit your intake of liquid calories
If you enjoy drinking sugar-sweetened beverages like soda, tea, juice, or wine, you may easily consume hundreds of calories per day. This means that they are "empty calories" because they provide more energy but no nutritional benefits.
Unless they are drinking a smoothie to replace a meal, you must make every effort to stick to water, unsweetened tea, or coffee. Water can be flavored with freshly squeezed lemon or orange juice.

Dehydration and hunger should not be confused. Drinking water regularly between scheduled meals helps sate an individual's appetite.

5. Keep an eye on portion sizes and totals
Even low-calorie vegetables may cause weight gain when you exercise, so always watch your diet.

As a result, it's wise to steer clear of portion measurements and to avoid eating food straight from the container. Using measuring cups and rules for serving sizes is the preferable option. Guessing causes overestimation, which increases the risk of eating too much food.

When eating out, use the following size comparisons to keep track of your food intake:
A golf ball is equivalent to 1/4 of a cup.
Half of a cup is occupied by a tennis ball.
Each cup holds one baseball.
One ounce (oz) is equal to a loose handful of nuts.
One playing die is equivalent to one teaspoon.
One tablespoon equals one thumb tip.
3 ounces of meat equals one deck of cards.
The only item is a DVD.
In the absence of the necessary tools, even though these measurements are approximate, they can still be utilized to assist someone in controlling their food consumption.

6. Conscious eating
It offers several advantages to eating with full awareness of one's why, how, when, where, and what one is eating.
Making healthy food decisions is directly impacted by gaining a greater understanding of the body.

Additionally, conscious diners try to chew their food fully and concentrate on the flavor. The body can perceive all satiety signals when a meal lasts 20 minutes.

It's important to bear in mind that feeling satisfied rather than full after eating is more important, and that many "all-natural" or low-fat foods aren't always a good choice.

Additionally, when choosing a meal, people can consider the following factors:
Does the "value" of the calories you eat seem to be fair?
Will it satisfy your hunger?
Are the components nutritious?
If there is any, what is the sodium and fat content?

7. Management of cues and stimuli
Many societal and environmental cues could encourage unnecessary eating. For instance, some people tend to eat too much when they watch television. It is challenging for people to pass a dish of candy to another person without munching on it first.

By becoming aware of what can make them want to munch on empty calories, people can come up with methods to change their routines to limit these triggers.

8. Take initiative

If a kitchen is equipped with foods that are ideal for diets and meal plans are created, weight loss will be more noticeable.

Get rid of all processed and junk food from your kitchen and make sure you have everything you need to make quick, healthful meals. In this way, you can control your weight loss. It's possible to prevent impulsive, hasty, and reckless eating by doing this.

Making meal decisions before attending social events or eating out could make the process easier.

9. Look for social aid

Being loved by people is a great way to stay motivated.

Accepting the help of loved ones is a necessary step in a successful weight loss quest.

Others could want to invite friends or family to join them instead of updating others on their progress via social media.

Additional sources of help could include:

Workplace assistance programs, a strong social network, individual or group treatment, fitness groups, or partners

10. Have optimism
If the pounds do not start to drop as quickly as you had thought, you could get discouraged because weight loss is a gradual process.
There will be days when sticking to a weight reduction or maintenance program is harder than others. Successful weight loss requires persistence and a refusal to give up, even when making changes in oneself seems unattainable.

Some people might need to rethink their goals by altering their workout regimens or the total number of calories they want to consume.

The secret to successfully conquering these challenges is to maintain a positive attitude and persevere in your efforts.

Losing weight: To successfully lose weight, it's not required to follow a strict eating plan like Slimming World or the Atkins diet. People should concentrate on consuming fewer calories and moving more to create a negative energy balance.

The primary determinant of whether or not someone loses weight is calorie restriction, not altering the ratios of carbohydrates, fats, and proteins in the diet. To start experiencing health benefits, a weight loss goal of 5–10% over six months is reasonable. The vast majority of individuals may achieve this goal by keeping their daily calorie consumption between 1,000 and 1,600. Less than 1,000 calories per day won't provide enough nutrition each day.

After six months of dieting, the rate of weight loss frequently decreases and the body weight tends to plateau as a result of people consuming less energy at a lower body weight. The simplest way to stop yourself from regaining lost weight is to adhere to a weight-management plan that includes a balanced diet and frequent exercise.

For people with a BMI of 30 or above who don't have any health problems related to obesity, prescription weight-loss medications may be helpful. Those with obesity-related diseases who

have a BMI of 27 or higher might also benefit from these.
Drugs should only be used, though, in conjunction with the aforementioned lifestyle adjustments. If weight loss efforts are unsuccessful and a person has a BMI of 40 or more, surgical therapy may be an option.

Chapter 2

REDUCE HIP AND ABDOMINAL FAT

GETTING RID OF BELLY FAT

A person may develop belly fat for several reasons, including poor diet, inactivity, and stress. By making dietary changes, stepping up their exercise regimens, and adopting a healthier lifestyle, people can lose belly fat.

Belly fat is a term used to describe abdominal fat. Two types of abdominal fat exist:
An individual's internal organs are encased with visceral fat.
Underneath the skin is where subcutaneous fat is found.

Subcutaneous fat has less of a detrimental effect on health than visceral fat.
People can change several factors of their food and lifestyle to lose belly fat.

Why is belly fat dangerous?

Being overweight is a major contributor to serious illnesses.
If you have too much abdominal fat, you run the risk of:
cardiovascular disease cardiac arrests
I have high blood pressure.
stroke
glucose type 2
bronchitis breast cancer
dementia caused by diarrhea

Causes of belly fat
These are typical reasons why people have too much belly fat:
1. A poor diet
Just a few examples of sweet foods and beverages are fruit juice, cakes, and candy.

cause weight gain to reduce metabolism and fat-burning potential

Low-protein, high-carb diets may have an impact on weight loss as well. Lean protein helps people feel fuller for longer, so those who don't consume it may eat more overall.

Trans fat in particular can be a factor in both inflammation and obesity. Trans fats are included in many products, especially fast food and baked goods like muffins and crackers.

According to sources, trans fats should be replaced by whole-grain foods, monounsaturated fats, and polyunsaturated fats.

Reading the food labels can help one determine whether it includes trans fats.

2. Alcohol abuse

Alcoholism in excess can cause inflammation and damage to the liver, among other health problems. Men who drink excessively tend to gain weight around their midsections, according to a poll on alcohol intake and obesity, however, female participants' results differed.

3. Lack of exercise

If a person consumes more calories than they burn off, they will gain weight.

Losing excess weight is difficult when leading an inactive lifestyle, especially in the abdomen.

4. Pressure

The steroid hormone cortisol is used by the body to manage and control stress. The body releases the hormone cortisol, which has an impact on metabolism when a person is in a hazardous or stressful situation.

A lot of people prefer turning to food as a solution when they feel restless. Cortisol stores these excess calories for later use in the area of the body near the abdomen and other areas of the body.

5. Transmission

There is some evidence that suggests a person's genes may have an impact on whether they become obese. Genes may impact behavior, metabolism, and the risk of developing fat-related disorders, according to scientists.

Environmental and behavioral variables might also affect a person's chance of becoming obese.

6. Insufficient sleep
According to a reputable source, insufficient sleep is connected to weight increase, which may lead to excess belly fat. However, the inference of causality is not permitted by this study.
Short sleep duration is linked to increased food intake, which could help belly fat develop. Potentially dangerous eating behaviors like emotional eating could come from not obtaining enough restorative sleep.

7. Smoking
Although smoking may not be a direct cause of belly obesity, scientists do think it is a risk factor. Smokers had more visceral and abdominal fat than nonsmokers, even though both groups' obesity rates were the same.

Achieving abdominal fat loss
The following actions may be beneficial for those who desire to lose belly fat:
1. Improving their nutrition
Eating a healthy, balanced diet can help someone lose weight and possibly enhance their general health.

Sugar, oily foods, and refined carbohydrates with little nutritional value may all be avoided. They can substitute a lot of fresh veggies, lean meat, and complex carbohydrates in its stead.

2. Reducing alcohol consumption
If someone wishes to lose their extra belly fat, they can control their alcohol intake. Sugar is regularly added to alcoholic beverages, which can lead to weight gain.

3. Increased exercise.
One of the many serious health problems that can arise from a sedentary lifestyle is weight gain. Everyone who wants to reduce weight should incorporate a reasonable amount of exercise into their daily routine.
Exercise that combines both strength training and cardiovascular activity can help people lose abdominal fat.

4. A rise in sunshine
A review found that animals exposed to sunlight might not grow as much weight or have aberrant metabolic processes.

The review found that few studies have looked at how sunshine impacts people's tendency to acquire weight, and more research is required.

5. Stress reduction
Stress can lead to weight gain. An individual's appetite may be impacted by the stress hormone cortisol's secretion, which could result in overeating. Yoga, and relaxation activities like mindfulness and meditation are methods for reducing stress.

6. Increasing the quality of your sleep
Health in general depends on sleep.
Even while a person's body needs sleep mostly to rest, recover, and heal, it can still have an impact on their weight.
It's imperative to get adequate sleep if you want to lose weight, especially belly fat.

7. Cessation of smoking
Smoking is undoubtedly harmful and increases the risk of developing belly fat as well as a host of other major health issues. However, you can decide to stop doing it to regain your general health and dramatically lower your risk of gaining too much belly fat.

Natural methods for abdominal fat reduction

Eat foods with few calories.
Select sugar-free beverages.
less sugar-filled carbohydrates
Fruits and vegetables
wholesome proteins
healthy fats
Exercise
more aerobic exercise
HIIT strength training
What triggers it?
Outlook

A person can lower their weight and body fat using tried-and-true natural methods by changing their diet and engaging in specific types of activity.

The sections that follow look at specific methods for losing belly fat.
1. Place a focus on low-calorie foods

One of the best ways to lose body fat is to consume fewer calories than what the body needs. This drives away fat from the whole body and also from the abdomen.

When one consumes fewer calories than what the body needs, this is known as a calorie deficit.

More often than not, foods with fewer calories are healthier than those with a lot of calories.

Consuming fewer foods that are high in calories but low in nutrition, such as processed foods, baked goods, and french fries, is a sensible way to create a calorie deficit and improve health.

In their place, choose wholesome, low-calorie foods like fruits, vegetables, lentils, and whole grains.

2. Eliminate sugary beverages.

The ingestion of extra sugar seems to be a significant factor in weight growth, especially in the abdomen.

Consuming a lot of sugar can increase visceral fat by causing insulin resistance and systemic inflammation.

It could be simple to drink sugar-heavy beverages without noticing it. Check the sugar content of beverages like soda-sweetened tea and coffee.

By avoiding soda and reducing the amount of sugar in hot beverages, many people can reduce the amount of added sugar in their diets.

3. Cut back on processed carbohydrates.
Refined carbs are high in calories but offer little in the way of nutrients. These carbs can be found in sweet foods and beverages, white bread, and refined grains.
Research has also connected refined carbs to reputable sources for information on abdominal fat gain.
Think about switching from processed to complex carbs. Fruits, vegetables, and whole-grain foods include them.

4. Eat more fruits and veggies.
Fruits and vegetables include complex carbohydrates, a nutritious, low-calorie alternative to processed carbohydrates.
Fruits and vegetables also contribute fiber to the diet. Fiber can help regulate blood sugar levels and lessen the risk of type 2 diabetes, a condition linked to the buildup of visceral fat and obesity, claims ResearchTrusted Source.

5. Pick lean proteins.
Lean protein can be found in nuts, lentils, and lean meats. These can be incorporated into a diet to encourage feeling satisfied after meals and reduce the desire for sweet snacks.
It can also be advantageous to consume less or no fatty foods, such as processed and beef meats.

6. Choose healthy fats
There must be some dietary fat in a healthy diet, however, not all fats are beneficial.
Saturated and trans fats can injure the heart, raising the risk of heart disease and stroke. They can lead to weight gain and are directly associated with the development of visceral fat.
Choosing healthy fats, on the other hand, can help you accomplish several benefits while also reducing your overall body fat.

Among the good high-fat options are:
Avocados and chia seeds
eggs, olives, fatty seafood, nuts, and nut butter
Learn more about the wholesome meals that are high in fat here.

7. Make an exercise schedule.

Exercise-induced weight loss can have an impact on every part of the body, including the belly.

It is impossible to completely get rid of fat in one area. This means that some exercises, such as crunches and sit-ups, may not always help you lose belly fat faster than others.

However, by engaging in these exercises, you may assist your abdominal muscles to become stronger and more defined.

8. Boost all-around activity

Expanding action levels throughout the whole day encourages calorie burning. Exercise can also help you gain muscle and feel better.

The following are some suggestions for increasing daily activity:

Sitting for long periods, taking frequent breaks for stretching, using a standing desk, parking further away, or taking the elevator in place of driving, cycling, or taking public transit.

9. Workout

The heart is stimulated by cardio, also referred to as cardiovascular activity. It also helps with weight loss and muscle toning by burning calories.

The cardiac exercises include:
using a bike to exercise while running
the water

10. Intervals of high-intensity training
High-intensity interval training (HIIT) involves
alternating periods of intense exercise with slower-
paced activities to burn calories.

For illustration, HIIT can consist of a cycle that
alternates between 3 minutes of walking and 30
seconds of running.

HIIT may have a greater ability to reduce body fat
than other types of exercise.
Due to the short durations, HIIT may also be a great
strategy to ease into a fitness routine.

11. Practice weightlifting.
Strength training can aid in weight loss because it
emphasizes building muscle mass, which burns
more calories than fat does.

Strength training can also improve the health of your
bones and joints. To support stronger muscles,

which are better able to support the body, the bones and joints won't have to work as hard.
While belly fat is common, having too much of it might be harmful. People who regularly eat processed and sugary foods are more likely to develop high levels of visceral fat.

REDUCE HIP ADIPOSITY.

Test One of These 10 Exercise Suggestions
Losing hip fat may be possible with the right diet and frequent exercise. Because it's difficult to target-reduce fat in just one section of your body, you must concentrate on losing weight throughout your entire body.
If your lower body is stronger and has less fat, your hips may appear smaller and more contoured. Additionally, having more muscle and being slimmer can increase your metabolism, making it easier to maintain a healthy weight.

The moment you realize there is a deduction in your weight, focus on exercises that will help tone the muscles in and around your hips and core.

Optional workouts and exercises
1. Squats
Squats are a versatile exercise that trains a range of muscles in the lower body. It's just easily done with body weight.
Once you've gotten the hang of it, you can make it more challenging by squatting down while holding a dumbbell or a kettlebell in each hand.
You can better complete a squat by standing with your feet slightly wider than shoulder-width apart. When executing bodyweight squats, you can balance yourself by holding your arms out in front of you. Engage your core, keep your back straight, and lower yourself until your thighs are parallel to the floor.
When your knees are slightly above but not quite over your toes, stop.
Exhale one more while standing up.
Count to 10 and 15 minutes

2. moves to the side.

A variation of the forward lunge is the side lunge, commonly referred to as a lateral lunge. It focuses more on the area of the hip and outside thigh.
As you stand, spread your feet just beyond hip-width apart. Step right with a big stride, then squat down, keeping your body tall, your core firm, and your eyes forward.
The right thigh should be parallel to the ground as you lower your body.
Pause. After that, take a left-foot stride forward before returning to the center.
12 to 16 times, swapping sides each time, repeat.

3. Water fountains
The "fire hydrant" workout targets your glutes and hip region. You can maintain stability by using the muscles in your core. You might want to execute this exercise on a mat if you have knee issues.
Kneel with your feet hip-width apart, palms towards the ground, and knees and feet shoulder-width apart. Maintain your modest forward and downward gaze. Engaging your core, raise your right leg off the floor and rotate it up and out to the side. Never let your knee stop being bent throughout the process.
When you get to the top, pause before putting your leg back in the position it was in before.

Perform 10 reps with the right leg first, then repeat with the left.

4. Wall seated

Wall sits, also known as wall squats, are great for building stronger hips, thighs, and lower abdominal muscles. They can be effective weight loss exercises, core strengthening drills, and muscular endurance tests.

Stand up straight with your back against a wall and your legs a few inches from the wall.

When you sit in a position with your legs at a right angle to the wall, your hamstrings should be parallel to the floor.

Hold this position for 20 to 30 seconds. As your strength and fitness develop, try to achieve 1 minute. Resuming the original position, stand up.

5. A bounding stroll

The banded walk workout entails moving side to side for a certain number of steps while keeping a resistance band tight around your hips. It's an excellent exercise for strengthening your glutes and targeting your hips.

Choose a wide exercise band that is light enough to allow you to execute 10 repetitions in each direction

while providing enough resistance to train your lower body.
Widen your stance, slightly flex your knees, and encircle your ankles with the exercise band.
Move to the side without allowing your feet to touch.
You can return to your starting location by taking 10 steps forward and 10 steps backward.
Count twice or three.

6. Weighted step-ups
Step-ups work your glutes, hips, and thighs. They might also improve your balance and steadiness.
Stand with your feet about hip-width apart in front of a step or bench that is high while holding a dumbbell in each hand.
Step onto the bench with your right foot and drive your left leg up, maintaining the weights by your side.
Off the bench, take a step back, and lower your left leg.
Perform 10 to 15 reps with your leading right leg, then switch to your leading left leg and complete the same amount of reps.
Do this two to three times on each of the particular spots.

7. Side-lying leg raise

The side-lying leg raise is a hip-specific exercise that tones and strengthens the hips. Correct form is crucial for this exercise.

Using a yoga mat, lie on your right side.

Slowly raise the upper leg of your left leg as high as you can. Continue toe-pointing forward.

When you get to the top, pause before putting your leg back in the position it was in before. Be careful to keep your core engaged and pelvis stable.

Repeat 10 times on each side.

8. Squat jumps

The squat leap is an advanced plyometric exercise that combines the normal squat with a jump for power training.

In a basic squat, place your feet shoulder-width apart.

Maintaining your weight on your heels, squat until your thighs are parallel to the ground.

From here, explode upward and drop.

Once you've touched down, shift into a squatting stance. After your feet ' balls have first contacted the ground, gently land, shifting your weight back to your heels.

Repeat after 30 seconds, or after 10 to 12 repetitions.

9. Ascending stairs

By climbing stairs, you may tighten and tone your glutes and hips in addition to receiving fantastic cardiovascular exercise. If you have access to a set of bleachers or a multi-level parking garage, you can sprint or jog up and down the stairs.
Sprint or jog up the steps, then slowly make your way back down. Spend five minutes doing this. You can also use a Stairmaster or step mill machine at the gym to simulate stair climbing.

10. High-intensity, sporadic exercise

HIIT, sometimes referred to as cardio interval training, requires you to engage in quick bursts of intense exercise followed by a quick break.

According to a study, HIIT can help you burn through calories quickly and reduce body fat.

On the treadmill, sprinting hard for 30 seconds and then walking for 15 seconds can make up an HIIT workout. You can also do jump squats or burpees for 45 seconds, then break for 15 seconds. There are several options and variations for a HIIT workout.

Generally, doing A HIIT workout should only be for 10 to 30 minutes. Try to do HIIT workouts at least twice a week.

Alternative strategies for lowering hip fat

Exercise is a fantastic strategy to build lean muscle and decrease body fat. It's also among the finest methods for continuing to lose weight after weight reduction. However, if you want to maximize your overall weight loss, it's imperative to consider other lifestyle changes.

1. Consume a healthy diet.
For weight loss and hip slimming, eating a balanced diet is crucial. Maintain a diet that prioritizes whole foods throughout all food groups.
Watch your portion sizes and refrain from adding sugar to your food or beverages. Try to consume fewer calories daily than you burn.

2. Have a restful night's sleep.

The right amount of sleep each night may help your weight-loss attempts. Make it happen at least by giving yourself seven to nine hours of restful sleep each night.

3. Maintain your composure.
Although stress is a part of everyone's daily lives, research shows that excessive stress can have harmful impacts on our health, such as headaches, weight gain, and high blood pressure. Because of this, stress management is a crucial part of any program to lose weight.
You might wish to try yoga, meditation, or deep breathing exercises if you feel stressed frequently. Exercise has been shown to lower stress levels. Consult your doctor or therapist about stress reduction techniques.

Takeaway
While it is impossible to target the fat on your hips precisely, you can design a program that prioritizes fat loss while emphasizing lower-body strengthening exercises. Hips that are stronger and more defined may result.

Chapter 3:

DIET STRATEGY

What Dietary Habits Suit Your Body Type?

The proponents of this method claim that by exposing details about your hormones and metabolism, knowing your body type will help you figure out how well you handle carbohydrates and how much protein you need. Not to mention, it might help you decide whether strength training at the local CrossFit gym or, say, signing up for that 5K you've been eyeing will help you become the healthiest, most energized version of yourself.

According to some research, each body type may have distinct characteristics in terms of weight, fat, and muscle; however, there is little evidence to support dietary and exercise recommendations, so don't count on them to be a magical cure.

How Does the Body Type Diet Work?
You might not be getting the results you want despite eating healthily and exercising. Numerous people are engaging in exercise for the first time in their lives and are eating healthier than before, yet they are still not taking excellent care of their bodies.
Your body shares traits with different body types that can help you determine how much muscle or fat you typically have, how fast or slow your metabolism may be able to burn calories, and, as a result, how easy or difficult it may be for you to lose weight.

There isn't much research on how a person's somatotype could influence how they choose their activities and nutrition. However, information on variances in body composition is available. There were 63 men between the ages of 18 and 40 in one small research. The researchers found that those with long and thin bodies had less body fat, weighed less, and had less lean body mass than those with curvy or hourglass proportions. correct up arrow

In a more recent investigation, the three-day diet diaries of about 150 women over the age of 57 were analyzed. They concluded that nutrition, exercise, fluctuating weight, body mass index (BMI), and even the existence of diseases were all related to somatotype. Participants with an hourglass body and those who were lean and lanky had lower diastolic blood pressure than those with curved proportions. Women who are thin and lanky are more likely to be underweight. When researchers looked at how much protein people ingested, they found that those who were curvy consumed more of it, and those who were lean consumed the least.
You can establish more attainable goals and get pointed in the direction of healthy habits that will work best for your body by determining your dominant body type. If you follow the same routine as someone with a different body type, you won't get the same results. It can help to refocus your goals on what is practical for you.

Understanding Your Type Using Your Body Type

There are three basic types of body. Due to regular exercise, dietary habits, and even metabolic changes brought on by pregnancy and menopause, you might not immediately recognize your body type. You may now be more of a hybrid type due to the way you live and how your body has changed as a result.

Very helpful
Consider how your body appeared in your late teens or early twenties if you're unclear about where your physique falls on the spectrum. You'll gain some understanding of your body's more innate metabolic state as a result. Here are a few additional suggestions from Just Your Type to assist you in choosing your category.

The ectomorph has a long, lean body. Due to your smaller bone structure, your shoulders typically tend to be narrower than your hips. Over time, you could come to realize that you have trouble gaining weight. This variety frequently has a higher tolerance for carbohydrates.

Mesomorph, You have an hourglass shape, a medium frame, and more muscle than fat.

Endomorph You normally have more body fat than the other body types in this framework. Endomorph women may be described as curvaceous, whilst endomorph men may be described as stocky. Your thighs, hips, and midsection are usually areas of excess weight. Endomorphs should limit their carbohydrate intake because they may be more prone to developing insulin resistance. When cells can't effectively absorb glucose from your blood, your pancreas responds by creating more insulin, which is a characteristic of type 2 diabetes. correct up arrow

Ecto-Mesomorphs
This physique is slender and powerful.

Meso-Endomorphs
This person is strong even if they don't have the well-defined muscles of a football player. However, this physique is more typical than you might think, and it is not exclusive to football players. In a prior review, 774 people were found to have an

endomorph and mesomorph combination as their most common somatotype. correct up arrow

Ecto-Endomorphs This describes someone who is naturally thin but has gained weight due to a poor diet and insufficient activity

What Amount to Eat Based on Your Body Type
The majority of the items suggested for each diet are substantial, nutrient-dense sources of carbohydrates, protein, and healthy fats. The macronutrient proportions are where they differ, with some foods being better suited for different body types. For instance, because endomorphs are advised to have fewer carbohydrates, it's possible that they wouldn't eat oatmeal. They would pick a breakfast strong in protein, like eggs, instead.

A day-long sample menu for ectomorphs from Sample Food Menus for Each Body Type

When it comes to the macronutrients—carbs, protein, and fat—ectomorphs ingest a 45-35-20 ratio of each. This suggests you'll be consuming a diet with fewer calories than the other diets. This suggests you'll be eating a diet with a reasonable quantity of protein, less fat, and more carbohydrates than you would on the other diets.

Breakfast oatmeal with fruit and nuts

Shake with protein as a snack

Chicken and vinaigrette-topped lunch salad with a variety of chopped veggies on top.

Snacking on apples and almonds

Quinoa with grilled shrimp and broccoli for dinner

A Mesomorphs Sample Menu for One Day

A mesomorph will attempt to divide their calories fairly evenly among the macronutrients.

eggs scrambled on bread for breakfast

Fruit with a protein bar for a snack

Variously cut veggies, chickpeas, and the dressing of your choice in a salad for lunch.

Hummus and vegetables as a snack

endomorph should maintain a 20-40-40 calorie split between carbohydrates, protein, and fat to decrease body fat. Eat grains with lunch or dinner, depending on when you work out.

breakfast of eggs and spinach

An energy bar with protein

roasted turkey lettuce wraps for lunch.

Hummus and vegetables as a snack

Chicken, quinoa, and zucchini noodles for dinner

Having a Body Type-Specific Diet Has Benefits
Understanding your somatotype and where you fit
will help you choose the foods to eat that will best
feed your body if reducing weight is your goal. The
fact that the body type diet is healthy is another
advantage. It may also prevent you from attempting
more severe diets that, at best, won't be successful
and, at worst, might backfire.

However, there is still a prescribed eating plan.
Ectomorphs, for instance, are believed to thrive on a
higher-carbohydrate diet, therefore a ketogenic diet
with extremely low carbs may put them at risk for
failure. It's one of the reasons the most recent diet
won't always provide the same outcomes for you as
it did for your friend who attempted the same
program. Additionally, your ambitions will be given
a dose of realism. Although anyone can dramatically
alter their birth body type, it relies on how much
time and work they're willing to invest. Your current
goal of having defined abs might not be the best one.
It might not go well with your body adjusting to

your current efforts to achieve distinct abs, and that's good. Contrary to common belief, there is no "perfect" diet; rather, what matters is enhancing your health. Working with your body type can also help you "understand how to maximize your potential and not get frustrated by your limitations," which is another advantage. For instance, endomorphs frequently struggle with weight loss. Knowing this beforehand will help you be more prepared to put in the necessary effort or modify your diet (by lowering carbs) accordingly. Having an idea of your body type helps set realistic expectations because weight loss can sometimes be very frustrating.

Problems with the Body Type Diet

There isn't enough evidence, according to many experts, to justify a body-type diet. "Using your somatotype to define your diet" just hasn't been studied. The only body type that matters for your diet is whether you are an apple or a pear, not how easily you can lose weight (naturally slim ectomorphs and more muscular mesomorphs will likely have an easier time due to their supposedly healthier insulin function). "Pears" have larger hips and thighs than they do for their smaller waist. "Apples" have a larger midsection, which is related to a higher risk of metabolic syndrome, as defined by a waistline of more than 35 inches for women and 40 inches for men. proper up arrow "Compared to someone who carries weight more evenly throughout their body, you're probably less responsive to insulin when you carry weight around your midsection. Apple types would be advised to stay away from grains and starchy carbs while implementing this technique to improve insulin sensitivity. This is true regardless of how you would characterize yourself; even ectomorphs with larger bellies are susceptible to health issues. Additionally, keep in mind that many people don't fit neatly into a system of body types. The fact that not everyone fits into a particular somatotype is an exception, so this no longer qualifies as a rule. Science doesn't support the idea that you should exercise for your type enough. "It's unclear if you should do the opposite of your strengths to balance yourself out or pursue your strengths to make the most of them. How to train people according to various physical types is still unclear.

How to Exercise for Your Particular Body Type

The body type diet recommendations allow your somatotype to direct you toward the best workout in addition to food choices. However, this does not imply that you should be restricted. Although you may be good at these things, we don't want to stop people from engaging in activities they enjoy. Ectomorph Even though you might naturally gravitate toward endurance activities like jogging, incorporating resistance training (like weightlifting or bodyweight exercises) can help you develop toned, lean muscles and reduce your chance of injury. HIIT is beneficial because it develops your anaerobic and aerobic cardiovascular systems while also increasing your strength and muscular mass.

Mesomorph Sports that call for short bursts of strength and power (like soccer or hockey) seem to come naturally to you, and you tend to put on muscle easily. You can, however, also easily reach fitness plateaus. Remember that switching up your routines every few months, mixing up the intensity of your activities (such as HIIT training, sprints, or kickboxing), and avoiding plateaus are all ways to stay in the best possible shape. Endomorph Once your stamina and endurance improve, HIIT workouts are a great way to generate additional fat-burning that lasts long after your workouts.

Foods to Consume for Your Best Body

Nothing you eat will instantly make you feel and look younger. However, getting the correct nutrients over time can have an impact. Here is the lowdown on five superfoods that can aid in weight loss, improve heart health, and enhance the appearance of your skin. Just as it's been said "real beauty comes from the inside" it's naturally known. The same might be said for being in good health. You start to look and feel your best when you maintain a healthy diet, get regular exercise, get enough sleep, and learn effective stress management techniques, such as swapping a Netflix binge for a yoga session or a long run in the park.

Uncertain about where to begin? Welcome to the five foods listed below. It has been demonstrated that they can aid in weight loss, heart health, and the promotion of healthy, younger-looking skin when included in a balanced diet.

1. Oat is a superfood!
Oats outperformed other whole grains when it came to decreasing cholesterol. In one study, eating oats helps people reduce their waistlines and lose overall body fat, which is in line with research showing that the fiber in whole-grain oats makes you feel fuller for longer. Oats also contribute to the health of your skin by supplying it with minerals like copper, zinc, and niacin. Oats' soothing effects on the skin can be obtained without even eating them: Oats in various forms have been applied topically for generations to cure dry, irritated skin.

2. Wild Salmon
You've certainly heard for years that salmon, and wild salmon in particular, is a great fish for your health. Here is one of the causes: Salmon includes astaxanthin, a form of antioxidant that reduces cholesterol and protects against heart disease. Astaxanthin can battle UV damage and improve skin suppleness, making it a potential weapon against aging. Weekly consumption of omega-3-rich seafood, such as salmon, decreased the occurrence

of precancerous skin lesions by roughly 30%. Studies have shown that salmon can aid in weight loss and that its omega-3 fatty acids may reduce abdominal fat.

3. Blueberries

Thanks to their high antioxidant content, which is higher than that of nearly any other food, these delicious little gems have powerful heart-healthy benefits. A weekly intake of three servings of blueberries and strawberries was associated with a more than 30% lower risk of heart attack. Antioxidants included in blueberries can make your skin seem younger by preventing and reducing the effects of sun damage. You feel full after eating blueberries, which may encourage you to eat less and lose weight.

4. Avocados

Did you know that people who consume avocados tend to be healthier than those who don't? Researchers found that people who ate avocados regularly lost weight, had less belly fat, and had a considerably lower risk of developing metabolic syndrome—a cluster of symptoms that can lead to

diabetes and heart disease. They also typically consumed more fruits and vegetables. We bet they even had lovely skin because avocados are abundant in the vitamins C, E, and K, all of which are essential for the health of the skin.
Furthermore, the healthy fat found in avocados may help prevent wrinkles, while other nutrients may minimize UV damage.

5. Pecans
Indeed, walnuts are high in calories. Their nutritional status is also improving, though. Walnuts have the highest concentration of heart-healthy omega-3 ALA of any plant food. They include a lot of fiber and protein, both of which can help you lose weight. Walnuts can aid in weight loss by stimulating a part of the brain that helps control cravings. Do you desire younger-looking, healthier skin? Walnuts can help there as well because they include minerals like vitamin E, zinc, and selenium that nourish and protect as well as antioxidants that slow the aging process.

Chapter 4

LIVING A NORMAL LIFE AND KEEPING A HEALTHY WEIGHT

If you are struggling to shed extra pounds or keep them off, you are not alone. which is why it's crucial to maintain a healthy diet and body.

Therefore, maintaining a healthy weight and eating plan is more important than ever. It's crucial to have a healthy lifestyle if you want to enhance your quality of life, but with so many fad diets and exercise routines to try, it can be difficult to know how to get healthier.

Although it is never easy to lose weight, it is always worthwhile. Maintaining a healthy weight will improve the performance of your body and lower your risk of future disease and discomfort. The majority of quick weight-loss methods fail since they don't provide you the ability to keep the weight off, despite the alluring headlines on magazine covers and web adverts. There is no secret weight loss formula, but there are some things you can do to maintain a healthy lifestyle.

The following tips can help you stay at a healthy weight:
* Pay attention to portion sizes.
By taking smaller bites, you can prevent overeating while simultaneously allowing yourself to eat more of the typical items you like. Serving sizes are different from portion sizes.

Eat nutritious foods.
Eating foods high in calories and sugar can contribute to weight gain if you're not careful. Choose delightful, nutritious foods like fruits, vegetables, and whole grains. You don't have to give up your favorite foods to take care of your body; it's acceptable to indulge in a few cheat meals or cheat days now and then.

* Drink more water.
By staying hydrated, eating correctly, and exercising each day, you may keep your weight within a healthy range. According to the Obesity Society, drinking water frequently can help you lose weight over time and change your body fat percentage.

* Maintain a food diary.
Because many people are unaware of their daily caloric intake, it is imperative to measure and maintain a record of it. It's necessary to shorten down on more of the calories than you consume if you wish to lose weight.

* Exercise every day
Your body weight is influenced by how much energy you use and consume. To maintain your current body weight, you must expend the same amount of energy that you consume; but, to lose weight, you must expend more energy than you consume. Find a fitness routine that includes weight training and cardio. In addition to helping you lose weight, exercise also strengthens your heart, builds muscle, and supports healthy internal functions.

* Get more sleep

A regular schedule of getting enough sleep each night helps your body to recharge and get ready for the next day. People who regularly lack sleep tend to overeat to stay awake. Make time in your daily schedule to get enough rest. If you follow this advice, you'll be able to function better throughout the day and prevent overeating. If you have trouble sleeping, try body-calming exercises like yoga, reading, or stretching.

* Decide on and stick to an objective.
To accomplish any goal, you must be conscious of your current circumstances. Find out what your Body Mass Index (BMI) is, then develop a plan to keep it within a healthy range. If you require support, speak to your family doctor or another medical expert. It is preferable to start with simple, short-term goals that you are sure you can accomplish. By doing this, you will be able to reach your long-term goals.

A Well-Rounded Life
Physical wellness can be supported by a happy, healthy mind. A balanced lifestyle includes focusing on healthy routines, thinking positively, and lowering stress.

All people desire to lead happy and healthy lives. What good is it to put forth the effort to live a long, healthy life if you can't enjoy it? While adopting a healthy lifestyle that includes regular exercise and a nutritious diet is beneficial for you physically, a balanced lifestyle also involves looking after your mental and emotional well-being. And at the top of your list of priorities should be stress reduction. Living a Life of Balance: Making the Commitment To have a balanced life, you must take into account all facets of your life, including your relationships, career, and physical and emotional health.

Balanced Living: Putting in the Work To have a balanced life, you must take into account all facets of your life, including your relationships, career, and physical and emotional health. And not be too exhaustible with job and family obligations, but scheduling time for yourself is essential if you want to manage everything. As a result, commit to taking daily "you time" delights and give your body and mind a physical and mental recharge.

Living Balanced Can Boost Happiness and Creativity

When you're happy, your outlook on life improves, which makes it simpler for you to approach your tasks. Stress, on the other hand, can make it harder for you to enjoy life and may even be harmful to your health. According to a study, stress might hinder creative thinking as well.

Make time for self-care and indulge in your favorite creative activities to reduce stress:

Make time for relaxation once a week, and allot a brief period each day for rest.
To have a cup of coffee and some tranquility in the morning before other people awake, get up a bit earlier.
Try a new ethnic dish for supper, take a leisurely aromatherapy bath rather than a quick shower, study a new language, or listen to new music on the way to work to make your regular routines more pleasurable.
Spend some time each week learning a new skill or indulging in a hobby you enjoy; taking art lessons, in particular, is inspiring and satisfying. Instead of just snacking on lunch while working at your desk,

spend your lunch break doing something you enjoy, like taking a walk, going out, or reading a book.

Always laugh out loud. Your health will benefit from it, and it can:
Become less stressed and prevent illnesses
Enhance mental health
lower blood pressure
Improve your mood
Healthy Lifestyle: Enjoying It Exercise for Health
Avoid pushing yourself to work out because you won't likely stick with it if you do. Do something enjoyable and rewarding that you are looking forward to finishing rather than another task that you might be tempted to put off. Exercise is essential for lowering stress, so make time for it and motivate yourself to go by:
Include a lengthy, rigorous workout in your weekend plans. Visit the gym, or plan a fun activity like a hike, bike ride, golf outing, or tennis match. Getting up earlier to exercise before you start your day or fitting in a workout during your lunch break at work.
Put your workouts on your calendar just like you would other important activities, and write down your plan to boost your motivation.

Fix and Fit

Schedule Time for Healthy Eating for Balanced Living

With the right diet, your body will stay healthy, you'll have energy, and your mood will get better. Learning new cooking techniques and healthy food combinations is fun, and healthy cuisine can be tasty. Furthermore, preparing healthy meals doesn't need to take a lot of time:

Look up heart-healthy dishes online or get a guidebook that emphasizes quick and delicious cooking.
Purchase freshly prepared fruits and veggies so that you can get them right away.
Make a healthy plan for the following week and get all the necessary ingredients. You'll be able to resist the impulse to order pizza if you have a strategy. Everything in moderation is a maxim that is commonly used and for good cause. Enjoy, laugh, and live a healthy lifestyle since everything in moderation indicates that your life is in a good condition of equilibrium.

Chapter 5

INCREASING ENERGY

Self-care tips to combat fatigue

Fatigue is frequently brought on by stress, lack of sleep, a poor diet, and other factors of one's lifestyle. Utilize these self-help techniques to increase your energy.

If you experience fatigue, which is extreme exhaustion that is not relieved by rest and sleep, you may have an underlying medical condition.

Eat often to prevent weariness

If you want to maintain your energy levels throughout the day, eating regular meals and healthy snacks every three to four hours is preferable to eating a large meal less frequently.

Take action!
You could feel as though exercising is the furthest thing from your mind. But over time, regular exercise will help you feel less worn out and give you more energy.

After just one 15-minute walk, you'll feel more energized, and the benefits increase as you exercise more frequently.

Just a little exercise at first. Over weeks and months, gradually increase your weekly aerobic activity to the recommended 2 hours and 30 minutes, such as cycling or fast walking.

Gaining energy by shedding pounds

If your body is carrying additional weight, it could be exhausting. Additionally, it puts more stress on your heart, which could exhaust you. If you lose weight, you'll feel a lot more energized.

In addition to eating sensibly, increasing your level of activity and exercising is the best way to lose weight and keep it off.

Sleep peacefully
Many people don't get enough sleep to stay awake all day.

For better sleep, experts advise avoiding midday naps, going to bed and waking up at the same time each day, and relaxing before bed.
lowering tension will boost energy
Stress significantly depletes one's energy. Attempt to fill your day with relaxing activities.
This could be:
working out in a gym
Reading, listening to music, practicing yoga or tai chi, and socializing with friends
If you engage in some form of relaxation, your energy will rise.

Talk therapy helps with fatigue
There is some evidence that cognitive behavioral therapy (CBT) or counseling may help in the fight

against weariness or exhaustion brought on by stress, anxiety, or a depressed mood.

Get rid of the caffeine
It is advisable to quit drinking coffee if you feel fatigued. The best way to do this, it suggests, is to gradually stop all caffeinated beverages over three weeks.

Caffeine is present in:
coffee, tea, cola, and energy drinks, along with a few medications and herbal remedies.
Try to completely abstain from coffee for a month to see if you feel less exhausted.

Headaches can occur if you don't consume coffee. If this happens, cut back on your coffee intake more gradually.

fewer drinks are consumed
Even if a few glasses of wine in the evening can help you fall asleep, alcohol reduces the quality of your sleep. Even if you get an entire eight hours of sleep, you will still feel worn out the following day.

Limit your alcohol consumption before bed. As a result, you'll sleep better and have more vitality.

According to research, neither men nor women should regularly consume more than 14 units per week, which is equivalent to 10 small glasses of low-proof wine or 6 pints of beer with a typical ABV.

Every week, try to skip a few days of drinking. You'll have more energy if the water is greater. Being tired is occasionally merely an indication of minor dehydration. A glass of water is the remedy, especially following exercise.

Chapter 6

CONCLUSION

Let's hope that both the procedure and the results of your weight loss are positive and that your journey will genuinely wow you.

You can now move about more easily, are more flexible, have stopped snoring, and your blood pressure has returned to normal after losing the excess weight.

The thrills are always unique because you are now feeling fantastic, looking better, and fitting into clothes better, among other things.

Good luck!

Fix and Fit